THE COMPLETE GUT-SOOTHING SOUPS COOKBOOK

A Guide with Nourishing Recipes to Manage Your Gut Health

Copyright @ 2023 by **BREN HAN PHD**

TABLE OF CONTENT

PREFACE

I have been delving into the intricate realm of gut health for quite some time, immersing myself in a sea of information in pursuit of a solution to my wife persistent gut issues. Little did I anticipate that the answer would come in a form so commonplace yet profoundly transformative; the soup.

These everyday culinary staples, is often overlooked, turn out to be the unsung heroes in my journey to restoring my gut health. It was a moment of revelation, a realization that something as simple as a bowl of soup could hold the key to my gut problems.

Literally, we consume soups routinely, almost mindlessly, but witnessing their potential as more than mere sustenance was a paradigm shift. As I delved deeper into the therapeutic aspects of soups, I discovered a world where everyday ingredients transformed into powerful healers.

INTRODUCTION

Digestive diseases affect 60 million to 70 million Americans, ranging from gallstones and irritable bowel syndrome (IBS) to Crohn's disease and ulcerative colitis. Know that Gut-related issues span beyond your GI tract. Signs of an unhealthy gut may show up as Chronic pain, Mental health issues (such as depression and anxiety), Weight loss, Migraines, Diabetes, Insomnia, Inflammation, Fatigue or lethargy But it's not all bad news. Gut health may help predict diseases, provide protection and offer possible treatment.

The gastrointestinal system is the main "portal" for taking in and processing nutrients, but it also serves a communication center and disease fighter. From your nervous and immune systems to your mental health and digestive function, a healthy gut plays a pivotal role in your overall well-being. Also known as the digestive tract or gastrointestinal (GI) tract, the gut covers the parts of the body involved with food intake and output from top to bottom. This includes the mouth, esophagus, stomach, small intestine, pancreas, liver, gallbladder, colon and rectum. But when we talk about gut health, we're really talking about the bacteria in the microbiome, and the vast majority of the "microbiome magic" happens in your large intestine. Think of the microbiome as the environment inside the large intestine, specifically the trillions of bacteria that live there.

Our body has an important, symbiotic relationship with our microbiome: it takes in all these microorganisms, digests them and then produces other compounds that our body can use. So, while some of these bacteria are harmful to our health and others are beneficial, they both need to be there.

This cookbook teaches you how to soothe the bacteria in gut with soup and live healthily.

CHAPTER ONE

DIGESTIVE SYSTEM ANATOMY

Your digestive system allows you to utilize food from such diverse sources as meat from an animal and the roots of a plant, and utilize them as an energy source. Whether it is the ability to coordinate the chewing of food without injuring our tongue and lips or the propulsion of the food from the stomach into the duodenum while releasing the appropriate enzymes, our digestive system allows us to manage the process without much thought and often while performing other tasks.

The Mouth

The mouth is the entry point for food, but the digestive system often gets ready before the first piece of food even enters your mouth. Saliva is released by the salivary glands into our oral cavity when we smell food. Once the food enters the mouth, chewing (mastication) breaks food into smaller particles that can be more easily attacked by the enzymes in saliva.

Your teeth can perform a cutting as well as grinding function to accomplish this task. The tongue assists in mixing the food with the saliva and then the tongue and roof of the mouth (soft palate) help move the food along to the pharynx and esophagus.

The Pharynx and Esophagus

After the food leaves your mouth where do think it goes? You need to get the concept clear here; as the food leaves the mouth it typically enters a road know has the pharynx that leads to two pathways. From the pharynx there are two paths that the food bolus can take, including:

- The wrong path, which is down the windpipe into the lungs

- The correct path into the esophagus and then the stomach

The act of swallowing is a complex process that closes the windpipe (to protect our lungs) and moves food into the esophagus.

This process is mostly automatic (reflex) but it is also partially under our direct control. Once it enters the esophagus, food is moved down the esophagus and into your stomach.

The Stomach and Small Intestine

From glands that line the stomach, acid, and enzymes are secreted that continue the breakdown process of the food. The stomach muscles further mix the food. At the end of this process, the food you placed in your mouth has been transformed into a thick creamy fluid called chyme. This thick fluid is then pushed into the duodenum (the first part of the small intestine). With the help of enzymes from the pancreas and bile from the liver, further breakdown of the food occurs in the small intestine. The small intestine has three segments;

- The duodenum where he further breakdown of the food takes place.

- The next two parts of the small intestine (jejunum and ileum) are mostly responsible for the absorption of nutrients from processed food into the bloodstream through the walls of the intestine.

After the small intestine, the leftover waste leaves the upper gastrointestinal tract (upper GI tract) which is made up of everything above the large intestine, and moves into the large intestine or colon (the beginning of the lower GI tract).

The Colon, Rectum, and Anus

The role of the lower GI (gastrointestinal) tract is to solidify the waste product (by absorbing water), store the waste product until it can be evacuated (going to the bathroom), and help with the evacuation process. The large intestine (colon) has four parts ascending colon, Transverse colon, Descending colon and

Sigmoid colon. Is it getting complex? You need it! All together the colon is approximately 7 feet long and connects to the rectum. Here as in most other parts of the GI system, the waste product is moved along by peristalsis. As the waste product passes through the colon, water is absorbed and stool is formed.

HEALTHY DIET FOR THE DIGESTIVE SYSTEM

To maintain good health, including a healthy digestive system, it is important to follow a balanced healthy diet that includes a range of foods. It is also important to make lifestyle changes such as avoiding smoking and keeping active.

A healthy diet means a balanced diet. It involves eating a range of different foods, from a variety of food groups, in adequate portion sizes. There are five different food groups; starchy foods (bread, rice, pasta, potatoes, cereals); protein foods (meat, fish eggs, beans); dairy foods (milk, cheese and yogurt); fruits and vegetables; oils and spreads.

One single food group cannot provide everything needed for good health, choosing a variety of foods from each group can help achieve a healthy balanced diet. Starchy foods, vegetables and fruit should make up the bulk of meals. All of those contain the most fibre, which is an important part of a healthy diet.

Fibre is not just important for good gut health and functioning: it is also associated with a lower risk of cardiovascular disease, type 2 diabetes and bowel cancer.

Starchy foods should be eaten regularly and you should aim to include one portion with each meal. Where possible higher-fibre starchy foods, such as wholegrain versions of bread, rice, other grains (barley, oats, buckwheat, bulgur, etc.), and breakfast cereals, should be consumed. Beans and pulses, seeds and nuts are also good sources of fibre and can help increase the amount, as well as the variety, of fibre we consume. The recommendation is to eat 30 grams of fibre a day but most people only eat an average of 18 grams a day. It is advisable to increase the amount of fibre consumed gradually and to drink plenty of fluids.

There are different types of fibre and each type behaves differently in your gut. Some types of fibre help make your stool bigger and easier to pass, which might help avoid constipation. Other types of fibre are digested (broken down) by your gut bacteria, producing substances that can be beneficial to your gut health.

They might also produce gases, which can cause bloating. People respond differently to different types of fibre and it is worth noting that many foods contain more than one type of fibre. High-fibre foods are also beneficial because they have a lower glycaemic index. Glycaemic index is a measure of the rate at which certain foods cause blood sugar to rise after they have been eaten. High glycaemic index food such as sweets and white (refined) starchy foods release a lot of sugar quickly, which your body has to use up or else it gets stored as fat.

A certain amount of protein is needed and can be obtained from many different sources including beans, pulses, fish, eggs and meat. Protein should be eaten in moderation. To avoid excess fat choose lean meat or remove excess fat and remove the skin from chicken. Milk and dairy foods are a rich source of calcium. Calcium is needed for healthy bones and teeth and it is recommended to have three servings a day from this food group.

Only a small proportion of foods should be made up of fatty and sugary foods. To maintain a healthy diet and lifestyle, in addition to eating the correct foods, it is also important to be aware of other factors. These include:

- Maintaining a fluid intake at around two litres per day.

- Monitoring portion sizes.

- Minimising fizzy or sugary drinks, including fruit juice.

- Limiting alcohol intake to 14 weekly units for men and women.

- Avoiding or reducing intake of certain foods such as sweets, cakes, crisps, chocolate, processed meats. Aim for less than six grams of salt per day and try to avoid adding salt to food.

- Eating at least five portions of fruit and/or vegetables per day.

- Eating at least two portions of fish per week, one of which should be oily (eg mackerel, trout, sardines, kippers or fresh tuna).

- Replacing saturated fat with polyunsaturated or mono-unsaturated fat.

All of us have short-lived gut problems from time to time. For the most part this settles down by itself and should give no cause for concern. However you should see your doctor about:

- A sudden but persistent change in the pattern of how your bowels work

- Bleeding from the back passage

- Increasing heartburn, indigestion or stomach pain

- Losing weight unexpectedly

- Persistent vomiting

- Difficulty swallowing

All these are especially true if you have a family history of significant gut illness. You should also see your doctor if you have been taking a remedy obtain from a pharmacy for more than 2 weeks without experiencing any improvement to your symptoms.

PROBLEMS LEADING TO UNHEALTHY GUT

How is your gut health? This is a question we're fast finding is one worth asking ourselves as research continues to mount up on the very important role our good gut health plays in our overall health, and how an unhealthy gut can be linked to a wide range of health concerns. We may immediately think of bloating, food repeating on us and painful digestion when it comes to gut health, but new research shows connections between our gut obesity, mental health challenges, food sensitivities, skin health, energy and more! So, how do you know if an unhealthy gut applies to you?

Extremes of an unhealthy gut can show up as irritable bowel syndrome (IBS) or bloating or gas, but there are other lesser known signs to be aware of. Some of these signs you may have been experiencing for your whole life without realising they were related to your gut, or that there are ways to support and manage them, or even be rid of them!

Having a healthy gut can ensure that your body, mind and spirit are healthy. On the other hand, poor gut health can sabotage your physical health and even your mental health in some sneaky ways. What causes an unhealthy gut? And how do you know if you're gut health needs improvement? Here are symptoms that hint at your gut needing a little loving attention.

Symptoms of an Unhealthy Gut

When your gut is healthy, your gut microbiota is in balance. Your good gut bacteria keep the bad gut bacteria under control to keep you healthy. When everything is working the way it should be, your gut health may seem "out of sight, out of mind." But when something is wrong, you can feel it everywhere. There are a few unwanted symptoms of an unhealthy gut:

Bloating, Burping and Bad Breath

Bloating and food repeating on you and bad breath is a hallmark sign that something is up with our gut. Firstly, bloating and burping can happen for a number of reasons, but mostly it's the result of what and how we eat or drink. Bloating is a sign of excess gas in our digestive system. When we eat or drink and we don't have enough digestive enzymes in our stomach to break it down for further digestion, our food will 'repeat on us' in an attempt to add more digestive enzymes in and break it down again. It can also be related to a food intolerance.

When it comes to bad breath, this is more related to the balance of good and bad bacteria in our gut and this bad bacteria making home in our mouth. The technical term for chronic bad breath is halitosis. In most circumstances, halitosis stems from odour-inducing microbes that live in between our teeth, gums, and on our tongue. It can also be linked to bacteria found in gum disease. Having these 'bad bacteria' living in our mouth doesn't paint the most pleasant picture for us and is quite a motivator for getting rid of them!

Give your stomach acid levels a boost with some added digestive enzymes, apple cider vinegar or lemon water to help break down and digest your food. Also keep a food diary on what foods trigger bloating, food repeating on you and flatulence the most and start to avoid them. And to love your gut, add in probiotics to build a stronger microbiome for digestion, good breath and healthy bowel movements.

Constipation, Diarrhoea and Gas

Whether our bowels are 'all go', or we have a constant feeling of being constipated and 'clogged up', or it's a mix of all of the above, irregular bowel movements are a sure sign of an unhealthy gut. When our gut is healthy the 'perfect poop' should ideally be around 30cm long a day and a nice soft and long 'sausage' shape.

This is important because if we're passing food too quickly in our stools, we miss out on absorbing important nutrients from it, and if we're constipated and food stays in us too long, it can create toxicity in our body.

A lot of this is largely related to the diversity and health of our microbiome. When the microbiome is imbalanced - meaning we have too many 'bad' and not enough 'good' bacteria we can notice irregular bowel movements and sensations like diarrhoea and gas. The number and diversity of bacteria living inside your gut impact your overall health and wellness.

There are a few different ways you can support having the best bowel movements for your health or the 'perfect poop' but some quick wins is to start keeping a food diary, notice how certain foods affect your bowels. Stay hydrated and drink plenty of water. Eat probiotic rich foods and/or take a quality probiotic for a healthy microbiome and lower digestive system and add in digestive enzymes such as lemon water, apple cider vinegar or a digestive enzyme supplement to help break down your food.

Food Intolerances and Sensitivities

Food intolerances and sensitivities are often felt in our gut. When we eat certain foods we may feel immediately bloated or our bowels may suffer. Most common food intolerances include gluten, dairy, nuts and the nightshade family of foods. If you experience food intolerances, it is almost always a result of leaky gut syndrome.

Leaky gut syndrome is when your gut barrier is compromised, which is not ideal, as your gut barrier is the gatekeeper that decides what gets in and what stays out of our digestive systems. Anything that goes in the mouth and isn't digested will pass right out the other end. This is, in fact, one of the most important functions of the gut is to prevent foreign substances from entering the body and bloodstream.

When the intestinal barrier becomes permeable (which happens when the junctions of the gut lining separate) this is leaky gut syndrome. Large food protein molecules can then escape into the bloodstream.

Since these proteins don't belong outside of the digestive tract, the body activates an immune response and attacks them. This immune response shows up as food intolerances and sensitivities.

Common food intolerances include gluten and dairy and are a great place to start when testing avoiding foods to improve your unhealthy gut symptoms such as bloating or indigestion.

Skin Problems

Because poor skin health is often linked to inflammation, which primarily starts in the gut, nurturing our gut health and ultimately our 'beauty from the inside out' is a great place to start for glowy, healthy skin. A common sign of food intolerances is eczema.

The link between leaky gut and autoimmune conditions such as eczema is significant. When our body marks a molecule as foreign invader our immune system is activated and will attack it, trying to clear it out of the body.

To do this 'invaders' are passed to the lymphatic system where they will then be eliminated from the body as toxins.

If the lymphatic system is unable to process these toxins completely, it may try to eliminate them through the skin. This then causes many common skin conditions, such as acne, eczema and psoriasis.

Nurture your gut lining by drinking plenty of gut loving bone broth or taking a quality collagen product to reduce gut permeability and leaky gut syndrome. Topping this up with some anti-inflammatory omega 3 fatty acids, high in DHA/EPA will also help you soothe and heal the skin.

The gut is one of the places where the immune system meets lots of foreign objects. Not just food and nutrients (and some non-food items), but bacteria, viruses, fungi and parasites. So, it may be no surprise the gut is one of the main places where your immune system resides.

There are many cells in the gut that work to release immune factors affecting the whole body, and others that function only to protect the lining of the gut. Ways to boost your immune system by growing great bacteria includes;

Try fermented foods

Fermented foods are an easy way to increase the beneficial bacteria in our gut. Kombucha, kefir, sauerkraut, kimchi and yoghurt have all been shown to contain bacteria and yeasts that can help reduce inflammation and improve gut bacteria growth. Start off with a small amount, 1-2 tablespoons daily, and increase over time. If you are pregnant please see our advice on fermented foods and pregnancy.

Eat more fibre

Gut bacteria digest certain fibres to produce short-chain fatty acids (SCFA), which reduce inflammation and can affect how the immune system works by changing immune cells. Acetate, the main SCFA produced by gut bacteria after digesting the fibre found in fruit, vegetables, nuts and grains, reduces gut permeability (leaky gut). Butyrate, another SCFA, reduces inflammation, improves the movement of food through the gut and may help protect against colon cancer.

Choose your alcohol carefully

Alcohol can increase the growth of certain bacteria that potentially cause an increase in toxins in the gut. Alcohol can also increase leaky gut and inflammation. Spirits may do more gut damage than wine or beer, and the amount and frequency of alcohol intake definitely plays a part in the amount of gut damage seen.

Manage stress

Not only does stress influence your gut bacteria, growing more of certain types of bacteria has also been linked to higher risk of experiencing anxiety and depression. Managing your stress can be one step towards improving your gut health and immunity.

Mind that fat

A high-fat Western-style diet reduces a bacterium called Akkermansia muciniphila, which plays a part in reducing inflammation through changes to immune cells.

Subtract some additives

Emulsifiers are additives mixed with certain foods to stabilise them. Usually they're added to keep two liquids, that don't usually mix, together, for example combining vinegar and eggs with oil to make mayonnaise. Lecithin, which is naturally present in egg yolk, helps keep the vinegar and oil together. Sometimes chemicals are used as emulsifiers, and indications are that these types of emulsifiers can increase the permeability of the gut lining. Choosing whole foods and avoiding packet foods as much as possible will help to reduce your intake of emulsifiers.

Make omega-3 regular

Regular omega-3 fats from fish have been shown to be great for our gut bacteria and, as an anti-inflammatory, are well known to help prevent heart disease and ease the pain of arthritis. Now it seems omega-3s also work to reduce inflammation in the gut by encouraging or discouraging growth of certain bacteria.

THE GUT SYNDROME

The leaky gut syndrome is a rapidly growing condition that people from the world over are experiencing of late. Although problems begin with your digestive system if you have the leaky gut syndrome, it affects other aspects of your health as well. Your gut is lined by a wall, which is similar to a net with small holes in them. These small holes act as filters and enable the passage of certain substances only. It acts as a shield to keep out the bigger, harmful substances from entering your body.

When someone has a 'leaky gut', it means that the gut lining is damaged and cannot optimally function as a barrier any longer. The smaller holes become larger and allow harmful substances like gluten, bad bacteria, and undigested food particles to enter your system and cause considerable damage to health.

Causes

There are 4 main reasons for the leaky gut syndrome:

- Dysbiosis, or bacterial imbalance, is a leading cause of the leaky gut syndrome. It means an imbalance between helpful and harmful species of bacteria in your gastrointestinal tract

- Poor diet, comprising proteins found in unsprouted grains, sugar, genetically-modified foods (GMO), and dairy products.

- Prolonged exposure to stress, which can weaken your immune system and inhibits your body's ability to eliminate harmful bacteria and viruses, resulting in inflammation and leaky gut.

- Toxin overload, that can lead to the leaky gut syndrome. We come across more than 80,000 chemicals and other toxic substances on a daily basis. However, the main culprits are antibiotics, pesticides, aspirin, and contaminated tap water.

Signs and Symptoms

- Digestive system changes like bloating, diarrhoea, gas, or Irritable Bowel Syndrome. Read more here.

- Seasonal allergies or asthmatic symptoms.

- Hormonal imbalances like PCOS (Polycystic Ovary Syndrome) and PMS (Premenstrual Syndrome).

- Autoimmune diseases like Rheumatoid arthritis, Hashimoto's thyroiditis, lupus, psoriasis, or celiac disease.

- Chronic fatigue or fibromyalgia.

- Mental health issues like depression, anxiety, attention deficit disorder (ADD), and attention deficit hyperactivity disorder (ADHD).

- Skin conditions like acne, rosacea, or eczema.

- Candida overgrowth, which is a fungal infection in humans.

FOODS FOR GUT-HEALTH

There are a number of things you can do to manage symptoms of a leaky gut. There are certain foods to eat and avoid if you have this condition.

- Vegetables, roots, and tubers such as broccoli, carrots, brinjal, beetroots, spinach, ginger, mushrooms, potatoes, yams, and squash.

- Fruits such as grapes, bananas, coconut, papaya, lemons and limes, pineapples, oranges, and strawberries.

- Sprouted seeds like chia, flax, and sunflower.

- Gluten-free grains like amaranth, brown rice, and gluten-free oats.

- Healthy fats like avocado, coconut and almond oils.

- Fatty fish like salmon, tuna, and other omega-3 rich fish.

- Meats and eggs.

- Herbs and spices.

- Cultured dairy products like buttermilk and greek yoghurt.

- Soups and beverages like bone broth, coconut milk, teas, and nut-based milk and products.

- Raw nuts like peanuts and almonds.

Foods to Avoid

- Wheat-based products like bread, pasta, wheat flour, and couscous

- Gluten-rich grains like barley and oats

- Processed meats and cold cuts

- Baked products like cookies, pastries, and cakes

- Snacks like crackers and granola bars

- Junk food or fast food

- Dairy products like milk, cheese, and ice creams

- Artificial sweeteners

- Refined oil

- Sauces and dressings with soy, hoisin, teriyaki and the likes

- Alcohol and carbonated drinks

CHAPTER TWO

Miso Vegetable Soup

Total Time: 35 Minutes

Ingredients

- 2 cups plus 3 tablespoons water, divided

- 2 tablespoons white rice

- 2 cups frozen stir-fry vegetables

- 1 12-ounce package extra-firm silken tofu, cut into small cubes

- 2 tablespoons miso, (see Note)

- 2 scallions, thinly sliced

- 1 teaspoon rice vinegar, or to taste

- 1/2-1 teaspoon sugar, to taste

Directions

- Bring 2 cups water and rice to a boil in a large saucepan over high heat. Cover, reduce heat to a gentle simmer and cook until the rice is just tender, 12 to 15 minutes.

- Add stir-fry vegetables to the pot, increase heat to high and bring to a boil. Cook until the vegetables are heated through, stirring occasionally, 2 to 3 minutes. Add tofu and cook until heated through, about 2 minutes. Remove from the heat.

- Combine miso and the remaining 3 tablespoons water in a small bowl and stir to dissolve. Add the miso mixture, scallions, vinegar and sugar to the soup and stir to combine.

Kale, White Bean & Pasta Soup

Total Time: 55 Minutes

Ingredients

- 2 tablespoons extra-virgin olive oil

- 1 medium leek, thinly sliced

- 1 medium yellow onion, chopped

- 2 medium carrots, scrubbed and chopped

- 2 medium stalks celery, chopped

- 2 medium parsnips, peeled and chopped

- 3 cloves garlic, minced

- 1 teaspoon dried oregano

- 1 teaspoon salt

- ½ teaspoon ground pepper, plus more for garnish

- 1 large bunch curly kale, stemmed and roughly chopped

- 8 cups reduced-sodium vegetable broth or no-chicken broth

- 12 ounces whole-wheat farfalle pasta or elbow macaroni

- 2 (14-ounce) cans no-salt-added cannellini beans, rinsed, divided

- 1 cup water

- Chopped fresh flat-leaf parsley for garnish

Directions

- Heat oil in a large pot or Dutch oven over medium heat. Add leek; cook, stirring often, until very tender, about 10 minutes.

- Add onion, carrots, celery and parsnips; cook, stirring occasionally, until the vegetables are slightly tender, 6 to 8 minutes. Stir in garlic, oregano, salt and pepper; cook, undisturbed, until fragrant, about 1 minute.

- Add kale; cook, stirring often, until it's just starting to wilt, about 2 minutes. Pour in broth; bring to a boil over medium heat. Cover, reduce heat to medium-low and simmer, stirring occasionally, until the kale is tender, about 20 minutes.

- Meanwhile, bring a large pot of water to a boil over high heat. Cook pasta according to package directions. Drain and set aside.

- Mash half of the beans in a medium bowl with a fork or potato masher until a chunky paste forms. Stir the mashed beans, the remaining whole beans and 1 cup water into the soup. Cook over medium-high heat, undisturbed, until warmed through, about 5 minutes. Divide the pasta among 6 bowls; ladle the soup over the pasta. Garnish with parsley and additional pepper, if desired.

Total Time: 30 Minutes

Ingredients

- 3 tablespoons canola oil, divided

- 1 tablespoon garlic paste

- 2 teaspoons ginger paste

- 4 cups lower-sodium vegetable or no-chicken broth

- 2 cups kimchi, drained

- 2 cups classic coleslaw mix

- 1 (14 ounce) package extra-firm tofu, drained and cubed (3/4-inch)

- 5 medium scallions, cut into 1-inch pieces

- 1 tablespoon reduced-sodium soy sauce

- 4 large eggs

- 1 tablespoon toasted sesame oil

- 1 tablespoon toasted sesame seeds

Directions

- Heat 2 tablespoons canola oil in a medium Dutch oven over medium heat. Stir in garlic paste and ginger paste; cook, stirring constantly, until fragrant, about 1 minute. Stir in broth, kimchi and coleslaw mix; bring to a boil over high heat. Reduce heat to medium-low and add tofu, scallions and soy sauce; cook, stirring occasionally, until the tofu is heated through, about 5 minutes.

- Meanwhile, heat the remaining 1 tablespoon canola oil in a large nonstick skillet over medium-high heat. Crack eggs, 1 at a time, into the pan; cook to desired doneness, 1 1/2 to 2 minutes for a runny yolk and 3 1/2 to 4 minutes for a firmer yolk.

- Divide the soup among 4 bowls. Top each with a fried egg. Drizzle with sesame oil and top with sesame seeds.

Spring Green Soup with Chicken

Total Time: 40 Minutes

Ingredients

- 2 tablespoons extra-virgin olive oil

- 1 pound chicken tenders

- 2 medium leeks, white and light green parts only, thinly sliced

- 1 medium yellow onion, chopped

- 2 stalks celery, chopped

- 2 cloves garlic, minced

- 4 cups low-sodium chicken broth

- ¾ teaspoon salt

- ¾ teaspoon ground pepper, plus more for
  serving

- 1 bunch asparagus, cut into 1-inch pieces

- 1 (5 ounce) package baby spinach

- 1 cup packed fresh parsley leaves

- ¼ cup grated Parmesan cheese, plus more for
  serving

Directions

- Heat oil in a large pot over medium-high heat.
  Add chicken and cook, flipping once, until
  browned and cooked through, about 6
  minutes total. Transfer to a plate.

- Add leeks, onion and celery to the pot.
  Reduce heat to medium and cook, stirring
  occasionally and scraping up any browned bits,
  until very tender, 6 to 8 minutes. Add garlic
  and cook for 1 minute. Add broth, salt and
  pepper; bring to a boil over high heat. Reduce

heat to maintain a simmer, cover and cook for 5 minutes. Add asparagus and spinach; cook until the asparagus is tender, about 5 minutes more.

- Shred the chicken into bite-size pieces and add to the soup. Stir in parsley and Parmesan. Serve the soup topped with more pepper and Parmesan, if desired.

Cabbage & White Bean Soup

Total Time: 30 Minutes

Ingredients

- 2 tablespoons extra-virgin olive oil

- 4 cups chopped green cabbage

- 1½ cups sliced leek

- 1½ tablespoons finely chopped garlic

- 4 cups lower-sodium vegetable broth

- ½ teaspoon salt

- 1 (15 ounce) can no-salt-added white beans, rinsed

- 1 Parmesan rind (optional)

- 1 tablespoon white-wine vinegar

- ¼ cup pesto

Directions

- Heat oil in a large Dutch oven or large pot over medium-high heat. Add cabbage and leek; cook, stirring often, until softened but not browned, about 4 minutes. Add garlic; cook, stirring constantly, until fragrant, about 1 minute. Add broth, salt, beans and Parmesan rind, if using; increase heat to high and bring to a boil.

- Reduce heat to low to maintain a low simmer; cover and cook, undisturbed, until the cabbage is tender, about 10 minutes. Remove from heat and stir in vinegar. Remove and discard Parmesan rind, if using. Divide the soup among 4 bowls, and top with pesto.

Spring Onion Soup

Total Time: 35 Minutes

Ingredients

- 1 pound spring onions (a mix of spring or salad onions and green onions), greens attached

- 2 tablespoons extra virgin olive oil

- 1/2 teaspoon sea salt, plus more to taste

- Fresh ground white pepper

- 1 medium Yukon Gold potato chopped into 1/4-inch pieces (1 heaping cup)

- 1/2 cup dry white wine

- 1 quart low-sodium vegetable or chicken broth

- 3 cups young leafy greens (I used a mix of kale and arugula)

- 1/4 cup shaved Parmesan

- 4 - 5 chives or blades of onion grass, minced

- 1 green onion, sliced thin, for garnish

Directions

- Move rack to top of oven and set broiler to high. Shave just the roots from onions, leaving core intact so that onion layers stay in place. Halve or quarter any larger onions. Arrange on a broiler pan and slide into oven. Broil until edges begin to char and onions are tender but still have some bite, about 10 minutes.

- Meanwhile, set a Dutch oven or small stock pot over medium heat. Add olive oil, and when hot, add potatoes, 1/2 teaspoon sea salt, and a few twists pepper. Sauté potatoes until tender with crisp edges, about 7 - 10 minutes. Add white wine, stir 1 minute, and then add broth. Bring mixture to a boil, then turn heat to low. Taste and add sea salt as needed.

- Working carefully in batches, blend charred onions, broth and potato mixture, and greens until smooth. (I like this soup with some texture, so I blend until the texture is smooth but still flecked with bits of char.)

- Pour back into soup pot and warm over medium-low heat just until mixture starts to steam. Heating soup gently is the best way to maintain its emerald green hue.

- Ladle into bowls and garnish with shaved Parmesan, minced onion grass or chives, thinly slice green onions, and several twists white pepper.

Total Time: 1 Hour 25 Minutes

Ingredients

- 1 pound small red beets, peeled and quartered

- ½ pound large carrots, peeled and halved lengthwise

- 2 ½ teaspoons olive oil, divided

- ¼ teaspoon salt

- 1 ½ cups diced peeled apple

- ¾ cup chopped yellow onion

- ½ teaspoon garam masala

- 2 cups organic vegetable broth

- 2 cups water

- 1 ½ teaspoons fresh lemon juice

- ¾ cup plain 2% reduced-fat Greek yogurt

- ½ cup chopped walnuts, toasted

- ⅓ cup baby watercress

Directions

- Preheat oven to 425°.

- Line a rimmed baking sheet with parchment paper. Place beets and carrots in a bowl. Drizzle with 1 1/2 teaspoons oil; sprinkle with 1/4 teaspoon salt. Toss. Arrange the vegetables on prepared pan. Bake at 425° for 40 minutes or until tender, stirring once. Remove from oven; cool slightly. Cut beets and carrots into 1-inch pieces.

- Heat a Dutch oven over medium heat. Add remaining 1 teaspoon oil; swirl to coat. Add apple, onion, and garam masala to pan; cook 1 1/2 minutes. Add beet mixture, broth, and 2 cups water; bring to a boil. Reduce heat, and simmer for 30 minutes. Remove from heat, and let stand 15 minutes.

- Place half of the beet mixture in a blender, and blend until smooth. Pour soup into a bowl. Repeat. Stir in lemon juice. Ladle about 1 1/4 cups soup into each of 4 bowls; top each serving with 3 tablespoons yogurt, 2 tablespoons walnuts, and about 1 tablespoon watercress.

Mushroom Miso Soup

Total Time: 10 Minutes

Ingredients

- 2 c Mushrooms, 100g/3.5oz

- ½ c Green leaves, 30g/1oz

- 1½ teaspoon Dashi powder, 5g

- 3 c Water, 720ml

- 2 tablespoon Miso paste, 36g, 1.3oz

Directions

- Slice mushrooms and chop daikon leaves.

- Put the mushrooms, daikon leaves, dashi powder, and water in a saucepan, and bring to a boil on medium heat.

- Lower the heat and simmer for two minute.

- Turn off the heat, add miso (use a miso measuring whisk if you have it), and stir gently until it dissolves.

Creamy Roasted Cauliflower Soup

Total Time: 1 Hour 10 Minutes

Ingredients

- 1 large head cauliflower (about 2 pounds), cut into bite-size florets

- 3 tablespoons extra-virgin olive oil, divided

- Fine sea salt

- 1 medium red onion, chopped

- 2 cloves garlic, pressed or minced

- 4 cups (32 ounces) vegetable broth

- 2 tablespoons unsalted butter

- 1 tablespoon fresh lemon juice, or more if needed

- Scant ¼ teaspoon ground nutmeg

- For garnish: 2 tablespoons finely chopped fresh flat-leaf parsley, chives and/or green onions

Directions

- Preheat the oven to 425 degrees Fahrenheit. If desired, line a large, rimmed baking sheet with parchment paper for easy cleanup.

- On the baking sheet, toss the cauliflower with 2 tablespoons of the olive oil until lightly and evenly coated in oil. Arrange the cauliflower in a single layer and sprinkle lightly with salt. Bake until the cauliflower is tender and caramelized on the edges, 25 to 35 minutes, tossing halfway.

- Once the cauliflower is almost done, in a Dutch oven or soup pot, warm the remaining 1 tablespoon olive oil over medium heat until shimmering. Add the onion and ¼ teaspoon salt. Cook, stirring occasionally, until the onion is softened and turning translucent, 5 to 7 minutes.

- Add the garlic and cook, stirring constantly, until fragrant, about 30 seconds, then add the broth.

- Reserve 4 of the prettiest roasted cauliflower florets for garnish. Then transfer the remaining cauliflower to the pot. Increase the heat to medium-high and bring the mixture to a simmer, then reduce the heat as necessary to maintain a gentle simmer. Cook, stirring occasionally, for 20 minutes, to give the flavors time to meld.

- Once the soup is done cooking, remove the pot from the heat and let it cool for a few minutes. Then, carefully transfer the hot soup to a blender, working in batches if necessary. (Do not fill past the maximum fill line or the soup could overflow!)

- Add the butter and blend until smooth. Add the lemon juice and nutmeg and blend again. Add additional salt, to taste (I usually add another ¼ to ¾ teaspoon, depending on the broth). This soup tastes amazing once it's properly salted! You can also a little more lemon juice, if it needs more zing. Blend again.

- Top individual bowls of soup with 1 roasted cauliflower floret and a sprinkle of chopped parsley, green onion and/or chives. This soup keeps well in the refrigerator, covered, for about four days, or for several months in the freezer.

White Bean and Kale Soup

Total Time: 30 Minutes

Ingredients

- 2 tablespoons olive oil

- 1 small onion chopped

- 2 (15 ounce) cans cannellini beans drained and rinsed

- 4 cups chicken broth

- 2 cups water

- 2 cups kale stems removed and torn into 1" pieces

- Salt and freshly ground black pepper

Directions

- Heat the oil in a 3 quart saucepan over medium-high heat until shimmering. Add onion and cook until softened, about 5 minutes.

- Meanwhile, mash one can of beans in a small bowl. Add mashed beans, broth, and water to saucepan. Bring to a boil.

- Stir in remaining beans (left whole) and kale. Reduce heat, partially cover, and simmer about 20 minutes, until kale is tender. Season to taste with salt and pepper (I like 1 teaspoon salt and ½ teaspoon pepper).

Chicken Vegetable Soup

Total Time: 35 Minutes

Ingredients

- 1 tablespoon extra-virgin olive oil

- 1 yellow onion, chopped

- 3 carrots, chopped (about 1 cup)

- 3 celery stalks, chopped (about 1 cup)

- 2 garlic cloves, minced

- 1 teaspoon dried thyme

- 5 cups water

- 1 1/2 cups fresh or frozen green beans , cut into 1-inch pieces

- 1 pound boneless chicken breasts

- 1 tablespoon fine sea salt (I use Real Salt brand)

- 1/2 teaspoon ground black pepper

Optional Additions

- 1 (15 oz.) can chickpeas or white beans , drained and rinsed

- 1 pound potatoes, cut into ½-inch pieces

- Fresh lemon juice

- chopped parsley

Directions

- In a large pot with a lid, heat the olive oil over medium heat and saute the onion, carrots, and celery until softened, about 8 minutes. Add in the garlic and thyme, and stir for one more minute.

- Add in the water, green beans, chicken, salt, and pepper. Bring the liquid to a boil and then cover the pot and lower the heat so the soup can gently simmer for 15 minutes. (If you want to add potatoes or chickpeas, now is the time to do that, too.)

- Check on the chicken by lifting it out of the pot and testing it with a meat thermometer. When the temperature reaches 160°F, you can use the tongs to remove the chicken and let it rest for 5 to 10 minutes, so it can finish cooking and reach a safe internal temperature of 165°F.

- Use two forks to shred the chicken, or cut it into small, bite-sized pieces. Return the chicken back to the soup pot, and adjust any seasoning to taste. You can add 1 more cup of water, for extra broth, or add in a squeeze of lemon juice, to help brighten the flavor. Ladle the soup into bowls and garnish with freshly chopped parsley.

- Leftover soup can be stored in airtight container in the fridge for up to 4 days.

Cauliflower Soup with Turmeric and Cilantro Oil

Total Time: 30 Minutes

- **Ingredients**

- 2 tsp. ground turmeric

- 1 tsp. ground cumin

* ¼ tsp. ground coriander seeds

* ¼ tsp. crushed pepper flakes

* 1 tbsp. coconut oil or extra virgin olive oil

* 1 med. onion, diced

* 1 tbsp. garlic, minced

* 1 large organic cauliflower, (about 2 lbs.)

* 6 cups bone broth (or regular beef stock, or vegetable stock)

* ½-1 tsp. sea salt

* cilantro oil

* 1 cup cilantro leaves, minced

* 1 med. garlic clove, minced

* zest of 1 lemon

* 2 tbsp. lemon juice

* 5 tbsp. extra virgin olive oil

- sea salt and freshly ground pepper to taste

Directions

- Remove the leaves from the cauliflower then roughly chop the stem and the florets, set aside.

- In a medium pot, combine the spices and dry sauté (i.e., without any oil or fat) for a minute until fragrant, stirring occasionally so they do not burn.

- Next, add the oil and the chopped onion to the spice mixture and cook until the onion is softened. Add the garlic and sauté for a few minutes more.

- At this point, add the chopped cauliflower, the broth and the salt to the pot and simmer on medium heat for about 15 minutes or until the cauliflower stems are tender when pierced with a knife.

- To make the Cilantro oil: Mince the cilantro leaves finely and place them in a small bowl. Add the rest of the ingredients and mix well. Taste and adjust the seasoning.

- Let the soup cool for 5 minutes and then insert an immersion blender in the pot. Blend all ingredients until smooth. Alternatively, you can use a blender – you might need to blend the soup in batches. Taste and adjust the seasoning to your liking.

- Return to the pot and heat again, gently. Serve the soup with a drizzle of the Cilantro oil.

CONCLUSION

As the author of this narrative, I extend a heartfelt invitation to you, dear reader, to embrace the profound significance of gut health. It is not merely a component of wellness; it is the bedrock upon which vitality is built. From the vibrant dishes simmering in your kitchen to the choices that grace your plate, let the understanding of gut health be the compass guiding your journey toward holistic well-being.

In the subtlety of a well-crafted warmth of a comforting soup, we discover the power to nourish, heal, and rejuvenate. The gut, often overlooked, emerges as the compass pointing towards a life imbued with energy, resilience, and balance.